Hea

for Troubled Hearts

D0447321

Healing Thoughts
for Troubled Hearts

written by
Daniel Grippo

illustrated by
R.W. Alley

ONE
CARING
PLACE

Abbey Press

Text © 2004 by Daniel Grippo
Illustrations © 2004 by St. Meinrad Archabbey
Published by One Caring Place
Abbey Press
St. Meinrad, Indiana 47577

Library of Congress Catalog Number
2004105700

ISBN 978-0-87029-385-6

Printed in the United States of America

Foreword

Troubles come in all sizes and shapes, from deep grief or serious illness to fleeting worry or passing disappointment. Our troubles can leave us feeling alone and isolated, fearful and discouraged. But it doesn't have to be that way.

There are a number of ways to respond when trouble knocks at the door of your heart. There is much healing to be found—in nature, in others, in yourself. You can reach out, reach up, and look within for answers to your questions and balm for your pain. You can use your troubles to learn, to forgive, and to grow.

This friendly and supportive book is designed to help you lighten the load that weighs you down. It suggests a number of simple steps that can be used to ease the pain and promote healing and serenity. It is designed to give you options and ideas you may not have considered, so that the next time trouble comes knocking, you'll have new ways of responding.

1.

Your heart is troubled. At times, the hurt may be sudden and sharp. At other times, it may feel like a dull ache. It may come and go, or feel like it will never leave.

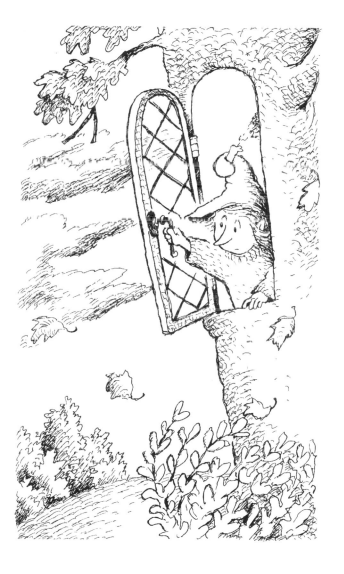

2.

Your heart may ache because a loved one has died. A loved one's death can leave a "hole" in your heart that feels like it will never heal.

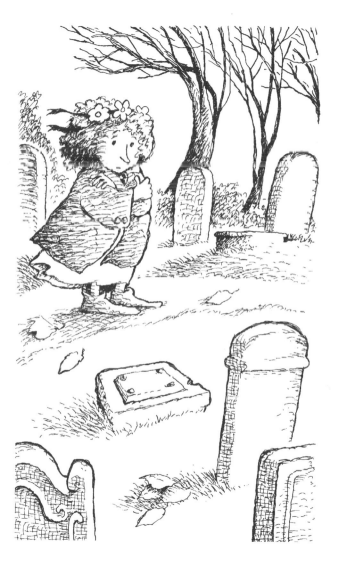

3.

Maybe you are troubled by an illness—your own or a loved one's. Serious illness leaves a person feeling isolated and afraid. It brings discomfort and limitations that can be hard to bear.

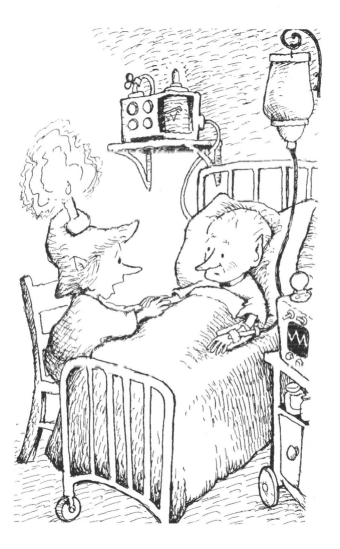

4.

Perhaps a relationship has ended, a loved one has left home, or you have recently been uprooted. Maybe you feel like no one is there for you. Loneliness and depression create a hurt that runs deep in the heart.

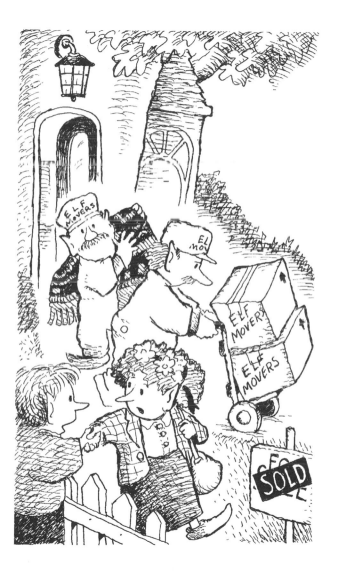

5.

Money worries, a job loss, an addiction or other personal struggle—any of these can leave you feeling anxious and insecure, casting a heavy shadow over your spirit.

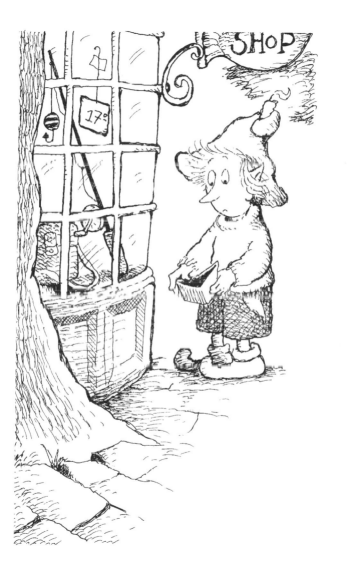

6.

Whatever the cause, your heart is troubled and you could use some support. But it's hard to know where to turn: "Who can I trust? Who will understand? How can I stop this ache in my heart? Where do I start?"

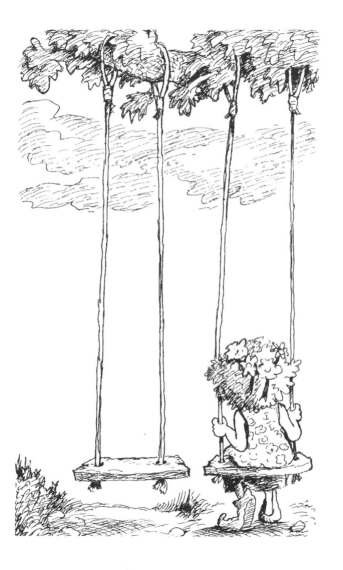

7.

Healing takes time. It doesn't happen in a day or a week. A troubled heart reacts like a hurting body—the deeper the wound, the longer it takes to heal.

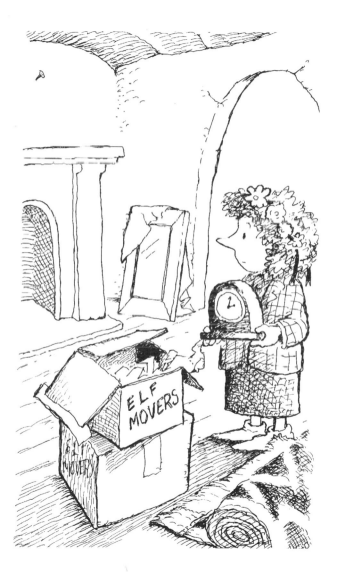

8.

Time won't erase your concern or loss, but it will bring some emotional distance. The hurt lives on, and at times will still feel painfully new. Be patient with yourself as you move through time with your pain.

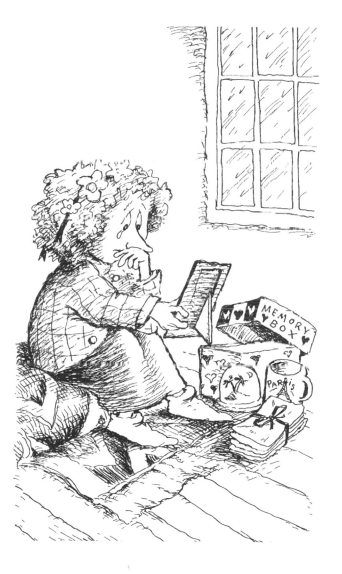

9.

Listen to the grief or worry in your heart. What is it saying to you? When does it hurt more? When does it hurt less? What seems to help ease the pain?

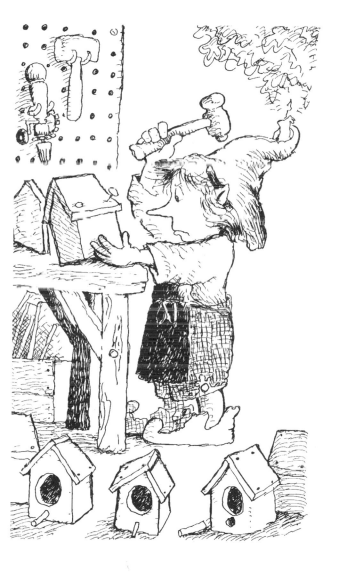

10.

Sometimes well-meaning loved ones tell us to "get over it" and "move on." While we do need to heal, it is also important to honor your feelings at this time. Don't allow yourself to be rushed.

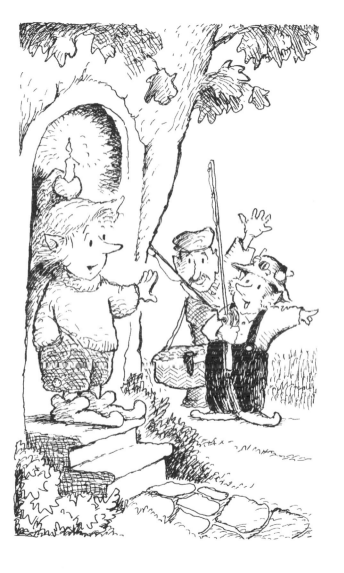

11.

Others can be supportive and helpful, but no one can tell you how, when, where, or for how long you need to feel these feelings. Give yourself permission to work through your troubles in your own way, in your own time.

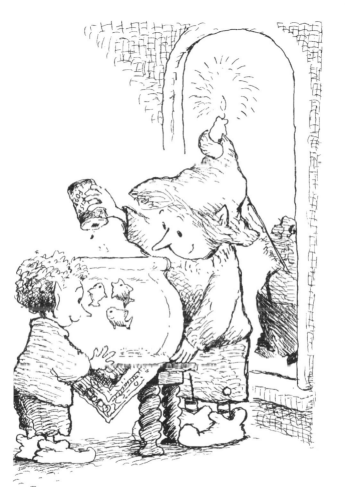

12.

Don't let anyone convince you that your grief or worry is a sign of weakness. It takes great strength to feel things fully. It is easier to numb yourself to the ache in your heart, but that will only delay your healing.

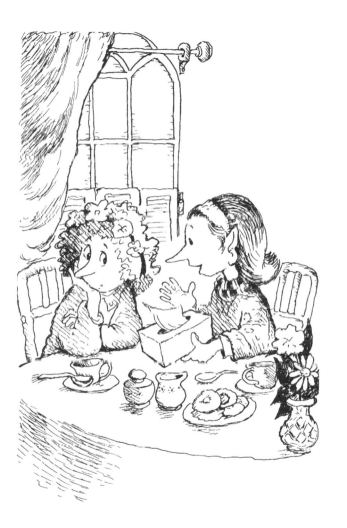

13.

As you feel the pain or worry, also try to analyze it. Tease apart the strands of your sadness or anxiety, and hold each strand up to the light. Ponder the many threads.

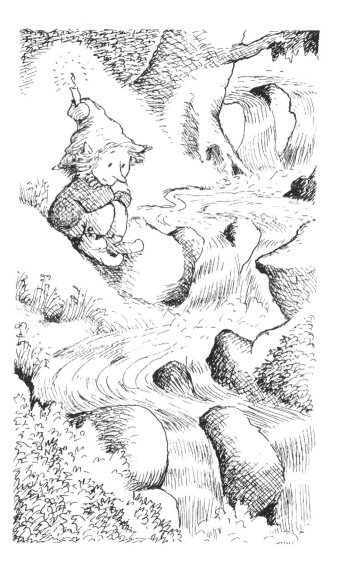

14.

Often, past and present hurts are mixed together in our hearts. You may have some unresolved losses or disappointments. Work through them one at a time.

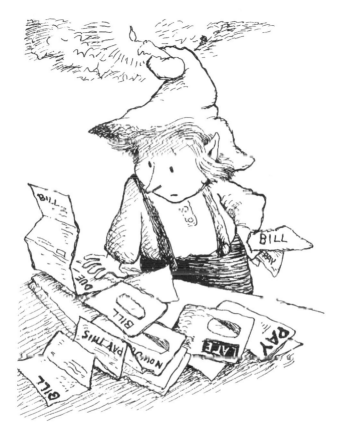

15.

Sometimes it's hard to get to the root of the pain. Talk with a friend. As you listen and share, you will find answers to some of the questions troubling your heart.

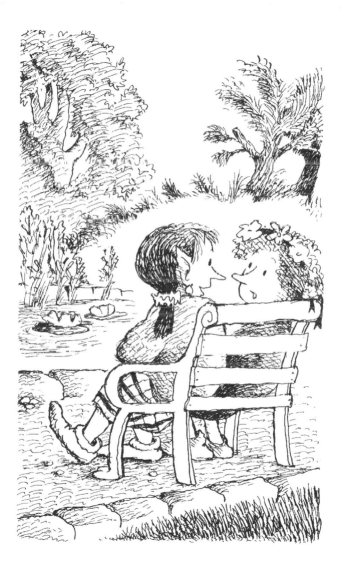

16.

There are many roads to healing. Each of us must walk our own path, but there are markers that can help us find our way. What activities serve to lift your spirits and boost your confidence? These will be your touchstones.

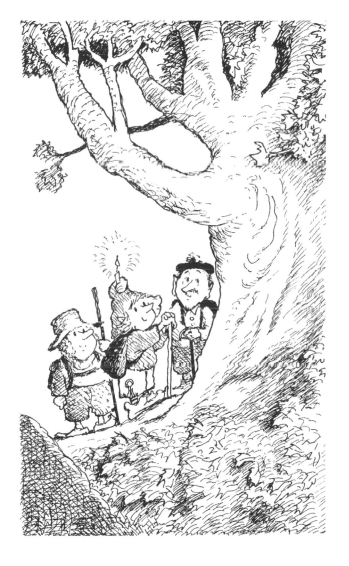

17.

Many people find that spending time with nature brings comfort. Tending a garden or walking in the woods can bring serenity and insight.

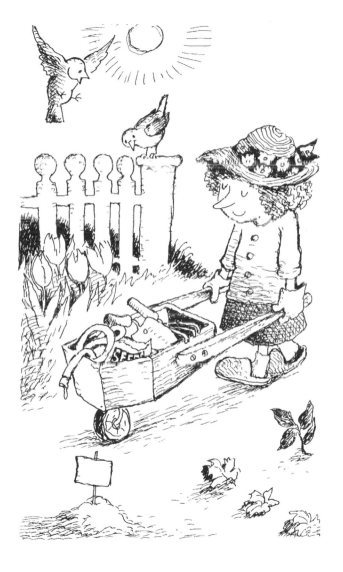

18.

Observe the coming and going of the seasons. While change is never easy or painless, it is a part of all creation.

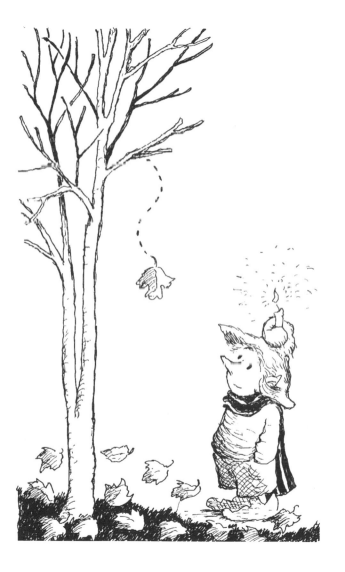

19.

Allow yourself to experience
the vastness of the ocean, the
majesty of a mountaintop,
the splendor of a sunset.
The universe is large enough
for your pain.

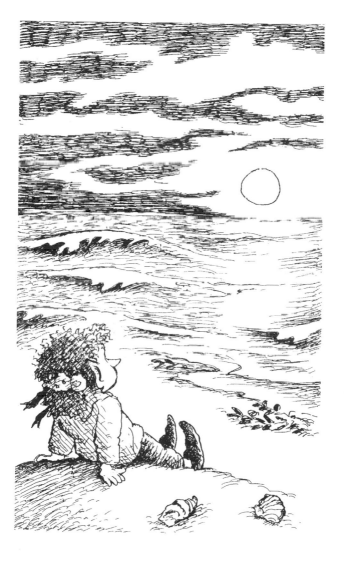

20.

Listen to your body. Where are the physical points of pain and tension? What could help bring relief? A massage? A warm bath? Treat your body well at this difficult time so it can help you heal.

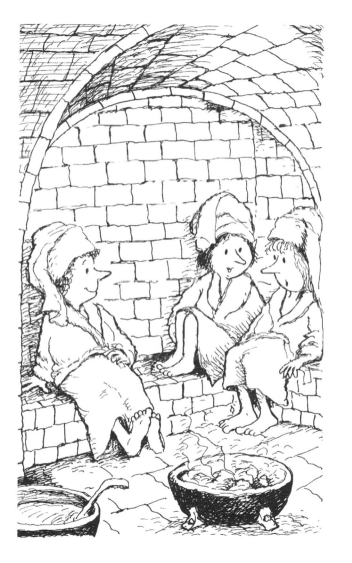

21.

Movement is helpful, especially when we are stressed or worried. Exercise elevates the spirit while releasing tension. An activity as simple as walking has great healing power.

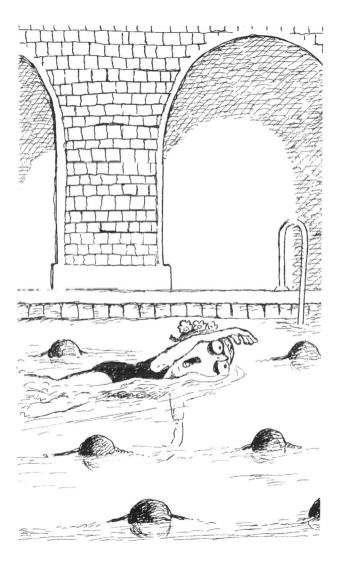

22.

Crying expresses and releases the pain you feel inside. It is one of the best things you can do when you hurt. Let the tears flow. They will help you heal.

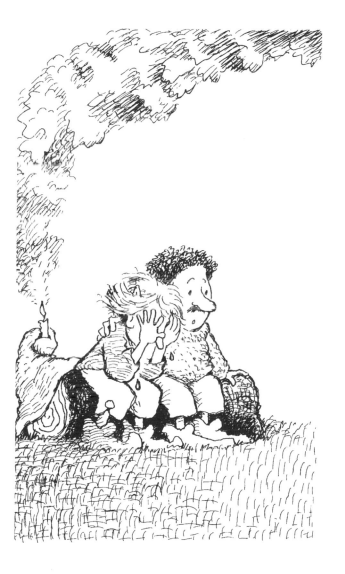

23.

Although you may feel all alone in your sadness or anxiety, there are others who have walked a similar path. A professional counselor or spiritual leader can help you connect with others and find support.

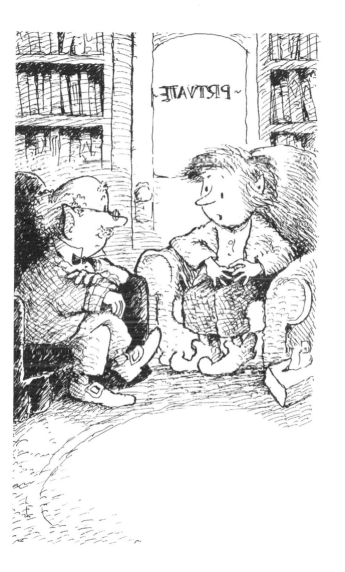

24.

Travel can refresh the spirit and provide new perspectives. Plan a trip to a place you've always wanted to see, or make plans to visit loved ones in another town.

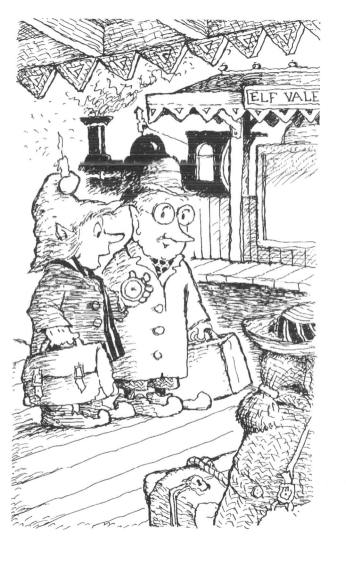

25.

A certain amount of solitude is helpful as you work through your troubles. But human companionship is also very important. Welcome solitude but avoid isolation.

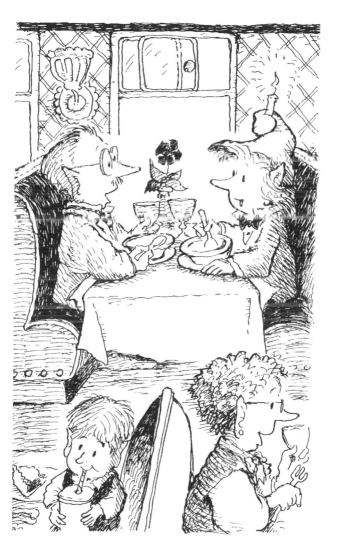

26.

The healing journey is also
a spiritual journey. Prayer,
reflection, and meditation
bring strength, insight, and
peace of mind.

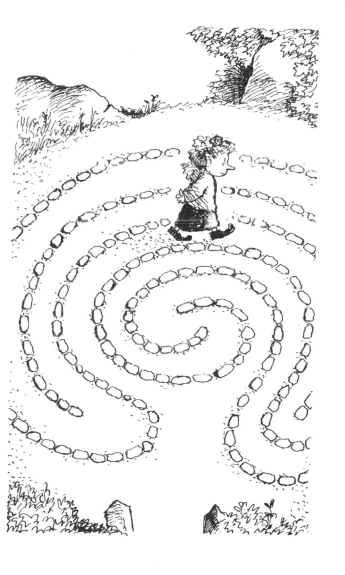

27.

Turn to members of your faith community for support when your heart is troubled. You will most assuredly find sympathy and solace. Remember, "In numbers, there is strength."

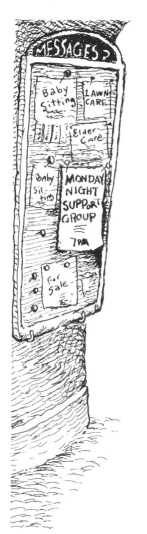
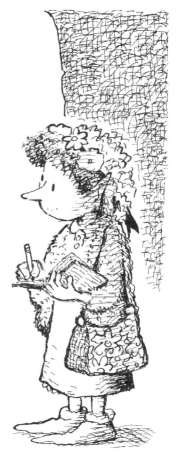

28.

Your suffering may seem pointless, until you realize that you can use it to connect with others in a compassionate way. Your pain can help you become aware of the suffering around you.

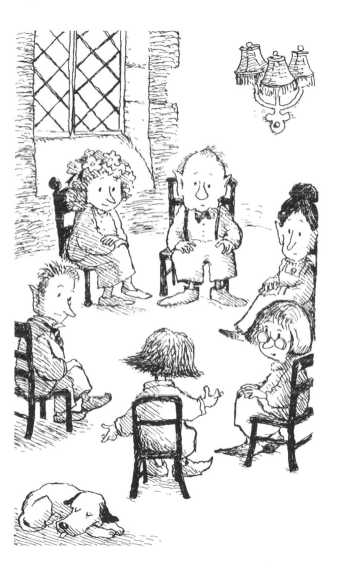

29.

Your troubles may suggest ways you can help others while helping yourself. For example, if you don't find a support group that suits your needs, start one at a local church, hospital, or funeral home. Turn your pain into something positive.

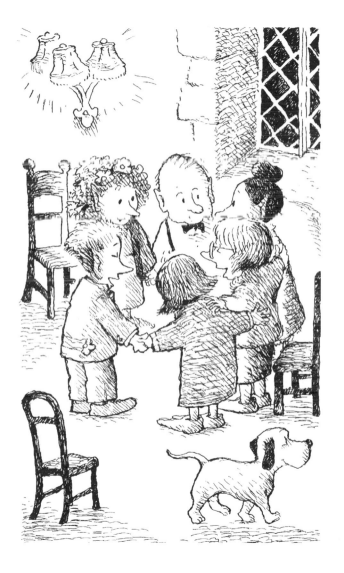

30.

"No pain, no gain" is a popular phrase among athletes, but it applies equally well to the spiritual life. Use your hurt to grow spiritually. Suffering can serve as a prod that motivates us to make needed changes.

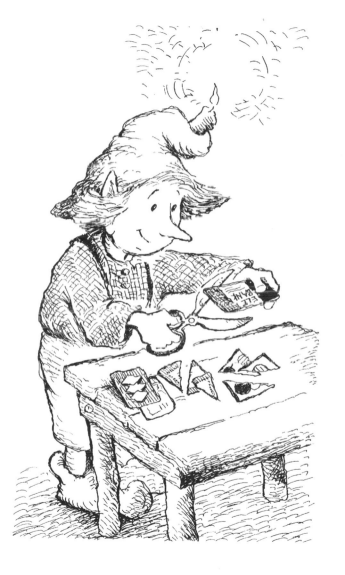

31.

Hope will help you heal. Make a list of all the things you hope for in the next three months. Hope creates the possibility of a brighter tomorrow.

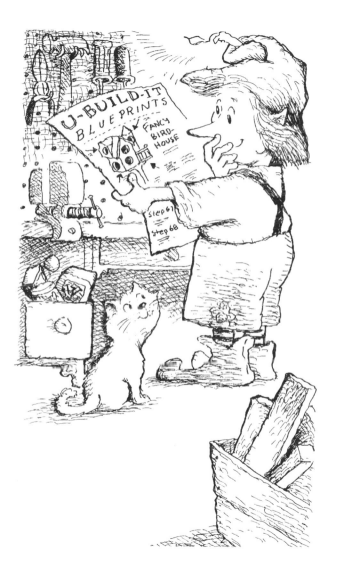

32.

Perhaps you need to forgive
someone who has hurt you.
It's difficult to do, but remember
that forgiveness blesses both
giver and receiver. Forgive
others so that you can be free
of resentment or bitterness.

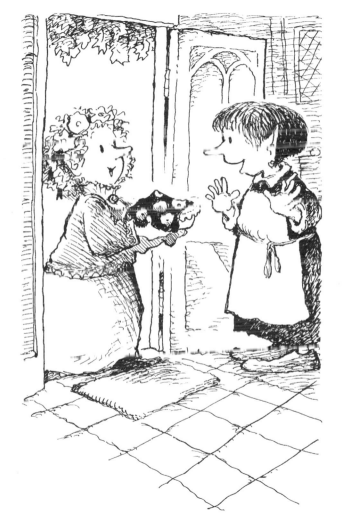

33.

Life brings its share of troubles, but healing comes from focusing on the good that remains: in you, in others, in the world around you. Indeed, "the light shines in the darkness, and the darkness does not overcome it." Focus on the light in your life.

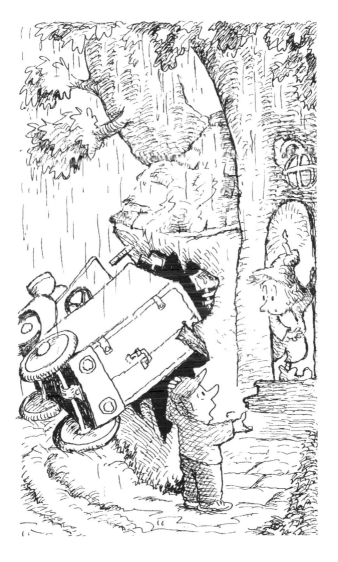

34.

An unexpected loss or upsetting turn of events can leave you filled with remorse. Realize that while you can't change the past, you can change the way you think about it.

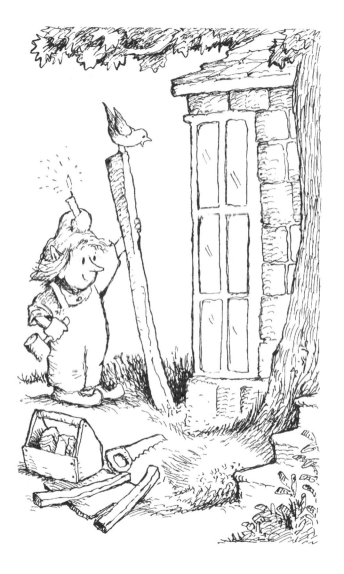

35.

Don't punish yourself for past mistakes. Glean the lessons that can be learned and apply them to your current circumstances. You will see that you have much goodness within you.

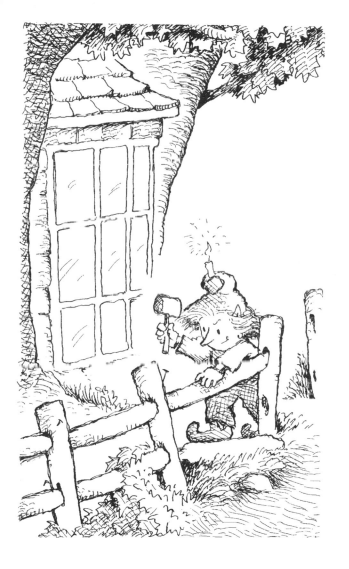

36.

Whatever the source of your troubles—grief, illness, loss, stress, change, anxiety—keep your mind focused on what you can do today to make things better. Don't let yourself be troubled by what tomorrow may (or may not!) bring.

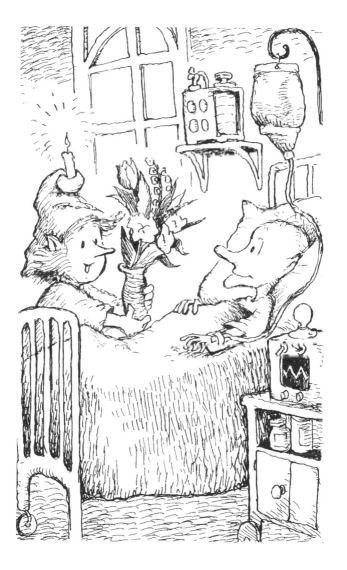

37.

One of the signs of healing is the ability to trust life again after a loss or setback. Start with small steps—invite a new friend into your life or take up a new interest. Life will respond to your trust with good things.

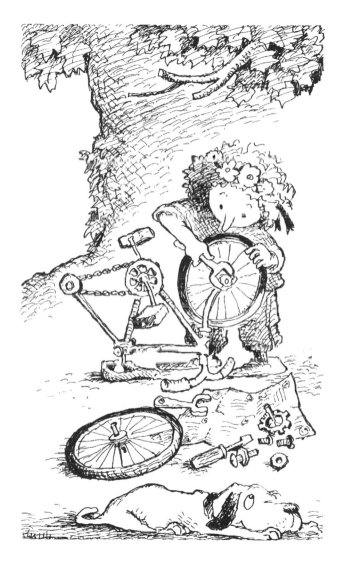

38.

As you journey toward peace and serenity, be gentle and patient with yourself, especially when progress seems slow. Do something special for yourself every day. And above all, trust that your heart will indeed sing again!

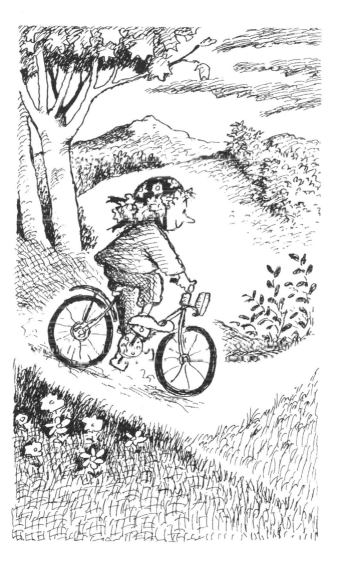

Daniel Grippo is a writer and editor of spirituality resources. He is the author of *Loneliness Therapy* (20078) and *Worry Therapy* (20093) from Abbey Press Publications. He can be reached at dgrippo@truequest.biz.

Illustrator for the Abbey Press Elf-help Books, **R.W. Alley** also illustrates and writes children's books. He lives in Barrington, Rhode Island, with his wife, daughter, and son. See a wide variety of his works at: www.rwalley.com.

The Story of the Abbey Press Elves

The engaging figures that populate the Abbey Press "elf-help" line of publications and products first appeared in 1987 on the pages of a small self-help book called *Be-good-to-yourself Therapy*. Shaped by the publishing staff's vision and defined in R.W. Alley's inventive illustrations, they lived out the author's gentle, self-nurturing advice with charm, poignancy, and humor.

Reader response was so enthusiastic that more Elf-help Books were soon under way, a still-growing series that has inspired a line of related gift products.

The especially endearing character featured in the early books—sporting a cap with a mood-changing candle in its peak—has since been joined by a spirited female elf with flowers in her hair.

These two exuberant, sensitive, resourceful, kindhearted, lovable sprites, along with their lively elfin community, reveal what's truly important as they offer messages of joy and wonder, playfulness and co-creation, wholeness and serenity, the miracle of life and the mystery of God's love.

With wisdom and whimsy, these little creatures with long noses demonstrate the elf-help way to a rich and fulfilling life.

Elf-help Books

...adding "a little character" and a lot
of help to self-help reading!

Book price is $4.95 unless otherwise noted.
Available at your favorite gift shop or bookstore—
or directly from One Caring Place, Abbey Press
Publications, St. Meinrad, IN 47577.
Or call 1-800-325-2511.
www.carenotes.com